Dietary Tips for Healing Uterine Fibroids and Hashimoto's Thyroidits

Including 40 Healing Recipes for Meals and Snacks

Dr. Aisha Steele Diallo

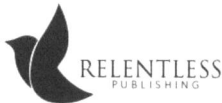

RELENTLESS
PUBLISHING

Published By :

Relentless Publishing House

RELENTLESS
PUBLISHING

ISBN : **978-1-948829-23-6**

First Edition : July 2019

10 9 8 7 6 5 4 3 2 1

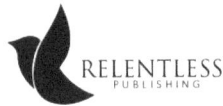

TABLE OF CONTENTS

Introduction

The human body is a complex network of organs and systems that all work together in harmony – at least that's how it should be. Unfortunately, there are many factors which can inhibit proper function of these organs and systems which can then have a negative impact on your overall health for both the short-term and the long-term.

Many of the body's major functions are controlled by chemical messengers known as hormones. Hormones are produced in the endocrine glands and they play a role in controlling basic human needs like hunger as well as more complex functions like reproduction. The endocrine glands are responsible for producing certain hormones, each of which has its own unique function. Some of the most important hormones in the human body are sex hormones which are produced by the ovaries in women and the testes in men.

In men, the testes produce testosterone, the primary male sex hormone (sometimes called an androgen) which is responsible for male characteristics that develop with the onset of puberty such as increased strength and muscle mass as well as facial hair growth. In women, the ovaries produce three sex hormones – estrogen, testosterone, and progesterone. Estrogen is the primary female sex hormone that regulates the menstrual cycle. Progesterone also plays a role in menstruation and pregnancy, particularly during the second half of the menstrual cycle. While it is completely natural for hormone levels to fluctuate to a certain degree, significant imbalances can lead to a variety of health problems – this is particularly true of the balance between estrogen and progesterone.

In this book, you'll learn all about estrogen dominance, a condition in which the body produces too much estrogen or fails to produce enough progesterone to balance it. You'll also learn about two related conditions – uterine fibroids and Hashimoto's thyroiditis – as well as some tips for using your diet to repair estrogen dominance. As an added bonus, you'll also receive 40 delicious recipes to help you reduce estrogen levels naturally.

Chapter 1: What is the Estrogen Dominance?

The ovaries are the main organs in the female reproductive system and they are responsible for producing both estrogen and progesterone.

What you may not realize is that estrogen is actually a class of hormones – there are three different types: estradiol, estrone, and estriol. These three estrogens work together at puberty to support the healthy development of female sex characteristics and to promote fertility. Estradiol is the primary hormone involved in breast development and fat distribution as well as the development of female reproductive organs.

Both estrogen and progesterone are involved in the process of menstruation and, while they are secreted by the ovaries, their release is triggered by another gland – the hypothalamus. Once a woman reaches puberty, the ovaries release a single egg each month in the process of ovulation and, as it migrates down the fallopian tube, a temporary gland in the ovary called the corpus luteum releases progesterone.

Progesterone triggers the lining of the uterine wall to

thicken in preparation for pregnancy. If the woman is not pregnant, the corpus luteum disappears and the lining of the uterine wall is shed. If the woman is pregnant, it triggers increased production of estrogen and progesterone which stops other eggs in the ovaries from maturing. The extra progesterone helps prevent uterine contractions which could inhibit the growth of the embryo. Near the end of pregnancy, estrogen levels rise which stimulates the pituitary gland to release oxytocin which triggers uterine contractions.

Balanced estrogen and progesterone levels are essential for healthy menstruation and for a woman's reproductive health in general. If the body produces too much or too little of either of these hormones, it can cause a variety of different problems.

When a woman's progesterone levels are too low, it is likely to cause abnormal menstrual cycles and could inhibit the woman's ability to conceive. Some signs of low progesterone levels include abnormal bleeding, irregular or missed periods, spotting, abdominal pain during pregnancy, and miscarriages. Low progesterone levels can also trigger excessively high estrogen levels, a condition sometimes referred to as estrogen dominance. Keep reading to learn more about this condition.

What is Estrogen Dominance?

In order to fulfill their intended functions efficiently, estrogen and progesterone need to be in balance. When estrogen levels are too high, it disrupts that balance and causes a condition known as estrogen dominance. The causes for estrogen dominance are many because there are numerous factors which can trigger increased production of estrogen or reduced progesterone secretion.

In some cases, estrogen dominance develops as a result of normal aging. Between the ages of 35 and 50, a woman's estrogen production decreases by about 35%. During that same period, her progesterone production drops by as much as 75%. Depending on the rate at which these hormones decrease, it could lead to an imbalance that triggers estrogen dominance. This is typically the age at which women begin to enter menopause, so symptoms are commonly linked to the menstrual cycle.

Aside from menopause, estrogen dominance can also be triggered by stress, allergies, obesity, impaired immune function, exposure to environmental toxins, improper diet, and concurrent medical problems such as autoimmune disease, breast or uterine cancer, and liver disease. Signs of estrogen dominance vary from one case to another but may include the following:

- Decreased sex drive
- Irregular or abnormal periods

- Water retention or bloating
- Breast swelling and tenderness
- Headaches or migraines
- Mood swings
- Weight gain (especially in hips and abdomen)
- Cold hands or feet
- Hair loss
- Problems with thyroid function
- Brain fog or memory loss
- Chronic fatigue
- Trouble falling or staying asleep

Though changing hormone levels are normal during a woman's menstrual cycle, excessive estrogen levels outside of this cycle is most commonly due to estrogen exposure in the food supply or the environment.

Environmental estrogens are divided into two categories: xenoestrogens and phytoestrogens. Estrogens that take the form of chemicals are called xenoestrogens and there are thousands of them – there are more than 70,000 registered chemicals in the U.S. that have been shown to have hormonal effects in addition to their toxic effects. Phytoestrogens are estrogens found in food and plants. Both phytoestrogens and xenoestrogens mimic the action of estrogen produced in the body and can alter your body's hormone balance and function.

While the negative effects of xenoestrogens are well

documented, they are still poorly understood. These chemical estrogens can increase the estrogen load in the body over a prolonged period of time, a problem compounded by the fact that they are difficult to detoxify through the liver. Xenoestrogens can be found in the following:

- Pesticides, herbicides, and fungicides
- Plastics made with BPA
- Beauty products made with parabens
- Fluoride and dental materials
- Nail polish and nail polish remover
- Fabric softeners
- Gas from copiers and printers
- Computer monitors with high EMFs

You may also be exposed to xenoestrogens if you microwave food in plastic containers or leave plastic containers out in the sun. Using organic and natural cosmetics, beauty products, and cleaning products can reduce your exposure to xenoestrogens as well.

Following a diet high in commercially raised meat, poultry, and fish can increase xenoestrogen levels in the body and contribute to estrogen dominance. This is because factory farmed animals like chicken, turkey, beef, and fish are often given estrogen-containing growth hormones to help them grow bigger and faster. Ingesting these animal products means that you're consuming those hormones as well.

Phytoestrogens are naturally occurring estrogenic compounds and they have a similar chemical structure to natural estrogen. When consumed through food products, phytoestrogens can change the production or breakdown of natural estrogen in the body or it could alter estrogen levels in the bloodstream. More than 300 food sources of phytoestrogens have been identified and are generally grouped into three classes:

- Isoflavonoids – These phytoestrogens are found in beans belonging to the legume family, primarily soybeans and soy products.
- Lignans – This type of phytoestrogen is commonly found in high-fiber foods like beans and cereal brans.
- Coumestans – These phytoestrogens are found in beans such as pinto beans, split peas, and lima beans as well as alfalfa and clover sprouts.

Being mindful of your everyday exposure to xenoestrogens and phytoestrogens can help reduce the risk for estrogen dominance but remember that there are many contributing factors. You'll learn more about a healthy diet to decrease estrogen dominance in Chapter 4.

How Does It Affect Men vs. Women?

While estrogen is a female sex hormone, it can be found in low levels in men as well – the same is true for testosterone in women. When a teenage boy reaches puberty, his testosterone levels will increase while his estrogen levels decrease. Later in life, testosterone levels begin to decrease while estrogen levels rise.

Not only is estrogen dominance in men a result of age-related hormone changes, but it can be linked to obesity and diabetes. Obesity is typically associated with an increase in body fat. Fat tissue contains an enzyme called aromatase which converts testosterone into estrogen – it also stores estradiol. Both of these factors contribute to increased estrogen levels in men. Estrogen dominance in men can also be triggered by excessive caffeine or alcohol intake and exposure to xenoestrogens and phytoestrogens.

Symptoms of estrogen dominance in men may be similar to those seen in women. Examples include decreased sex drive, weight gain or increased body fat, chronic fatigue, and emotional disturbances. Other symptoms may include enlarged breasts, benign prostatic hyperplasia (BPH), loss of muscle mass, and type 2 diabetes.

Dietary changes are generally the best option for reducing estrogen levels in men. Eating more cruciferous vegetables may increase estrogen detoxification, as can foods rich in vitamin B12, folate, betaine, and choline. Increasing fiber intake, exercising regularly, and reducing bodyweight may be beneficial as well.

Abnormally high estrogen levels can wreak havoc on your health, regardless whether you are male or female. In addition to causing a variety of negative symptoms, estrogen dominance can contribute to secondary health problems such as uterine fibroids and Hashimoto's thyroiditis, a form of hypothyroidism. Keep reading to learn more about each of these conditions and how to resolve them through dietary changes.

Chapter 2: Estrogen Dominance and Uterine Fibroids

While estrogen dominance is a condition that can affect both men and woman, only women develop uterine fibroids – the reasons should be obvious. Uterine fibroids are noncancerous growths of the uterus which typically appear during a women's childbearing years – they are also known as leiomyomas.

Though uterine fibroids can be linked to genetic factors and various growth factors, they are most commonly linked to hormonal changes – particularly, changes affecting estrogen and progesterone levels. Keep reading to learn more about what uterine fibroids are and how they are linked to estrogen dominance.

What Are Uterine Fibroids?

Noncancerous growths of the uterus are known as leiomyomas, or uterine fibroids. These growths are not inherently dangerous, and they are not associated with an increased risk of uterine cancer and they very rarely develop into cancer. Many women develop uterine fibroids at some point during their lives, but they are most common during the childbearing years.

While many women develop uterine fibroids during their life, most women don't show symptoms and therefore don't know that they have them. Fibroids are most commonly discovered by accident during routine pelvic exams and prenatal ultrasounds. Though most women don't develop symptoms, uterine fibroids can cause the following:

Heavy periods

Periods lasting more than a week

Pelvic pain or pressure

Frequent urination

Difficulty emptying the bladder

Constipation

Leg pain or backache

Doctors are not entirely sure what causes uterine fibroids, but genetic changes, growth factors, and hormone imbalance are likely involved. Risk factors for uterine fibroids include heredity, race, and environmental factors. Women who have an immediate family member with fibroids are at a higher risk for developing them, as are African American women. Environmental factors like early onset of menstruation, use of birth control, obesity, unhealthy diet, vitamin D deficiency, and alcohol consumption may also increase your risk.

Uterine fibroids are not inherently dangerous, but they can cause some discomfort and may lead to complications in rare cases. Anemia from heavy periods is one potential complication, as is infertility or loss of pregnancy. Fibroids can also increase the risk of pregnancy complications. Unfortunately, researchers have not discovered a way to prevent fibroids but maintaining a healthy body weight and eating a balanced diet may help you reduce your risk.

While the exact cause for uterine fibroids is unknown, a link has been demonstrated with estrogen dominance. Estrogen is the primary female sex hormone, so it makes sense that the main female reproductive organ – the uterus- is sensitive to estrogen. Fibroid growth is stimulated by estrogen and women who have estrogen dominance have a higher risk for fibroids.

Tips for Reducing Uterine Fibroids

Because uterine fibroids typically are not dangerous, treatment may not be required unless you are experiencing symptoms. In many cases, fibroids shrink over time and may disappear entirely after menopause when estrogen levels drop by 50%. When uterine fibroids cause discomfort and other symptoms, however, there are things you can do to reduce them.

One method for treating uterine fibroids involves application of progesterone cream to help restore the estrogen-progesterone balance. Natural progesterone creams have a low risk for side effects and they are very easy to apply.

Though progesterone cream can help balance progesterone levels in the short-term, long-term changes are your best bet for healing fibroids and preventing them from coming back. Maintaining a healthy body weight is important, but the best thing you can do is make changes to your diet to support hormonal balance. According to scientific research, the best diet for reducing estrogen levels is a low-fat, high-fiber, plant-based diet – this change is particularly effective when switching from a high-fat diet heavy in refined carbohydrates.

Here are some specific dietary recommendations which have been shown to help reduce uterine fibroids:

- Consume at least 30g dietary fiber per day
- Avoid high-glycemic foods including refined sugar and processed carbs
- Limit caffeine intake and alcohol consumption

- Eat plenty of cruciferous vegetables (like broccoli, cauliflower, and cabbage)
- Limit your intake of soy produces like tofu and edamame
- Take herbs to fortify the liver and speed estrogen clearance from the body
- Consume plenty of antioxidants, especially Vitamin C
- Get your recommended daily dose of beta-carotene, selenium, and zinc
- Drink at least 10 glasses of water a day to support detoxification

Making and maintaining these dietary changes are your best bet for balancing your estrogen levels and reducing uterine fibroids. Later in this book we'll go into greater depth about dietary recommendations to repair estrogen dominance.

Chapter 3: Understanding Hashimoto's Thyroiditis

Many doctors define estrogen dominance as an epidemic. Though the technical definition for epidemic is, "a widespread occurrence of an infectious disease in a community at a particular time," the CDC defines an epidemic as a sudden increase in the number of cases of a disease above what is normally expected. The alarming rate at which estrogen dominance is becoming increasingly common satisfies the criteria for this particular definition.

Another condition doctors often describe as an epidemic is hypothyroidism, or underactive thyroid gland. Hypothyroidism is a condition in which the thyroid gland fails to produce adequate levels of thyroid hormones. Keep reading to learn more about hypothyroidism, including one specific form of the disease.

Understanding the Thyroid and Hypothyroidism

The thyroid is a small gland in the neck that produces two specific hormones – triiodothyronine (T3) and thyroxine (T4). These hormones play a role in numerous bodily processes but mainly the metabolism. They control the rate at which the body utilizes fats and carbohydrates, regulate body temperature, and influence heart rate. When these hormones become imbalanced, it can lead to a number of symptoms including the following:

- Chronic fatigue
- Constipation
- Increased sensitivity to cold
- Dry skin
- Unexplained weight gain
- Hoarse voice
- Muscle weakness
- Puffy face
- Elevated cholesterol
- Muscle aches and tenderness
- Painful or stiff joints
- Heavy or irregular periods
- Slowed heart rate
- Thinning hair or hair loss
- Depression
- Impaired memory

If left untreated, hypothyroidism may progress, and these symptoms will worsen. When hypothyroidism becomes advanced, it can lead to a life-threatening condition known as myxedema.

There are numerous potential causes for hypothyroidism including autoimmune disease, thyroid surgery, radiation therapy, and certain medications. It can also happen when people with hyperthyroidism (overactive thyroid) are treated with anti-thyroid medications. Risk factors for hypothyroidism include sex, age, family history, autoimmune disease, thyroid surgery, pregnancy, and treatment with radioactive iodine or anti-thyroid medications.

Hypothyroidism affects women much more frequently than men – especially women over the age of 60. It is also closely related to estrogen levels in the body. Changing levels of reproductive hormones like estrogen can trigger hypothyroidism. The most common cause of hypothyroidism is a disease called Hashimoto's thyroiditis.

What is Hashimoto's Thyroiditis?

Research reveals that estrogen has a direct effect on the thyroid gland by impairing its ability to produce thyroid hormone, thus triggering hypothyroidism. What you may not realize is that there are different causes of hypothyroidism – Hashimoto's thyroiditis is one of the most common.

Hashimoto's thyroiditis is an autoimmune disease – it is a condition in which the immune system mistakenly attacks the thyroid gland, causing it to become inflamed and impairing its function. As is true for all autoimmune disorders, the exact cause for Hashimoto's is unknown. What research has revealed, however, is that certain things can trigger the disease to manifest – one of them is estrogen dominance.

This form of hypothyroidism affects about 5 out of every 10 people in the United States and it is about 8 times more common in women than men. In many cases, the first sign of a problem is the development of a swollen gland in the throat also known as a goiter. Over time, the disease can progress and produce other symptoms such as fatigue, changes in appetite or weight, trouble sleeping, joint and muscle pain, and dry skin. It can also cause changes in menstrual periods.

The most common treatment for Hashimoto's is hormone therapy involving synthetic thyroid hormone. In addition to hormone replacement therapy, there are certain diet and lifestyle changes you can make as well to help manage the condition. Here are a few recommendations:

- Avoid iodine supplements and limit your intake of iodine-rich foods
- Consider a plant-based diet to help the body detoxify and restore pH balance
- Eat foods rich in selenium such as eggs, legumes, brazil nuts, beef, and chicken
- Get your daily dose of zinc from shellfish, beef, chicken, legumes, and milk
- Remove gluten from your diet and consider cutting out processed grains

As you may notice, some of these recommendations overlap with dietary recommendations for reducing uterine fibroids from the previous chapter. In the next chapter, we'll go into greater depth about the proper diet to repair estrogen dominance and to relieve related conditions such as fibroids and Hashimoto's.

Chapter 4: Dietary Tips to Repair Estrogen Dominance

Estrogen dominance can affect both men and women. Because it typically involves an imbalance of estrogen and progesterone, simply supplementing with progesterone may not be the best treatment option. For long-lasting change, dietary changes are the best way to repair estrogen dominance. Keep reading to learn about these changes.

Good and Bad Foods to Repair Estrogen Dominance

Research shows that a plant-based diet is very beneficial for reducing estrogen levels and repairing estrogen dominance. If you aren't ready to make such a significant change to your lifestyle, however, you should at least be mindful of the kind of animal products you eat. Avoid factory-farmed animals because they are often treated with antibiotics and growth hormones – choose grass-fed, pasture-raised, and free-range meat and poultry as well as wild-caught fish and seafood instead.

In addition to being mindful of your meat intake, you should also focus on getting at least 30 grams of fiber per day. Your body excretes excess estrogen through the process of digestion but if you don't get enough fiber, you could become constipated and may reabsorb the estrogen your body was trying to get rid of. To meet your daily fiber needs, eat plenty of fresh fruits and vegetables, beans, legumes, nuts, and seeds.

Here are some of the best foods to eat to repair estrogen dominance:

- Grass-fed and pasture-raised meats
- Free-range poultry and cage-free eggs
- Wild-caught fish and seafood
- Leafy green vegetables
- Cruciferous vegetables like broccoli, cauliflower, and cabbage
- All varieties of mushrooms
- Foods rich in antioxidants like berries, green tea, nuts, and dark chocolate
- Resveratrol-rich foods like grapes, dark chocolate, and cranberries
- Polyphenol-rich foods like nuts and seeds
- Unrefined gluten-free grains like brown rice, quinoa, and oats
- Foods rich in vitamin B12 like fish, meat, poultry, eggs, and milk

- Natural sources of selenium like brazil nuts, tuna, halibut, turkey, and chicken
- Foods rich in zinc like wheat germ, spinach, pumpkin seeds, and beans

In terms of foods you should avoid to repair estrogen dominance, try to stay away from soy products like tofu, tempeh, and edamame because they contain isoflavones which can mimic the effects of estrogen and throw off your hormonal balance. It may also be a good idea to avoid processed grains and gluten as well as artificial additives like colors, flavors, and preservatives.

Though dietary changes are the best way to repair estrogen dominance for the long term, they should be paired with healthy lifestyle changes for maximum benefit. Do your best to lose excess body fat and maintain a healthy bodyweight. You should also get regular exercise, including strength training in your routine. Finally, learn how to manage and decrease your stress.

Tips for Avoiding Environmental Estrogens

In addition to making changes to your diet to repair estrogen dominance, you should also do your best to avoid environmental estrogens. Here are some simple tips for avoiding xenoestrogens and phytoestrogens:

- Do not purchase food or drinks in Styrofoam containers
- Don't heat foods and drinks in plastic containers and don't leave them in the sun
- Store food and beverages in glass or ceramic containers, not plastic
- Use organic or natural beauty and skin care products whenever possible
- Consider alternative birth control options – avoid birth control pills
- Use natural or organic cleaning and pest control products
- Don't buy factory-farmed meat treated with antibiotics and growth hormones

Now that you have a better idea what kind of diet to follow and how to avoid environmental estrogens, all that is left is to put that newfound knowledge into action. To get you started, you'll find forty delicious recipes in the next section that follow the dietary guidelines provided in this chapter. Enjoy!

Chapter 5: Recipes to Heal Fibroids and Hashimoto's

By now you have a thorough understanding of uterine fibroids and Hashimoto's as well as the common link that connects them – estrogen dominance. Reducing estrogen levels to restore your estrogen-progesterone balance is very important and it can be accomplished through making healthy and lasting changes to your diet.

In this chapter, you'll find a collection of forty recipes for breakfast, lunch, dinner, snacks, and desserts to help you lower your estrogen levels naturally and, in doing so, repair conditions like uterine fibroids and Hashimoto's as well as estrogen dominance. So, pick a recipe and give it a go!

Recipes Included in this Book:

Cucumber Spinach Dip

Black Bean Brownies

Cherry Chia Pudding

Avocado Chocolate Mousse

Cocoa-Dusted Almonds

Flourless Almond Butter Cookies

Gluten-Free Berry Crisp

Vegan Carrot Cake Cupcakes

Sweet Potato Breakfast Skillet

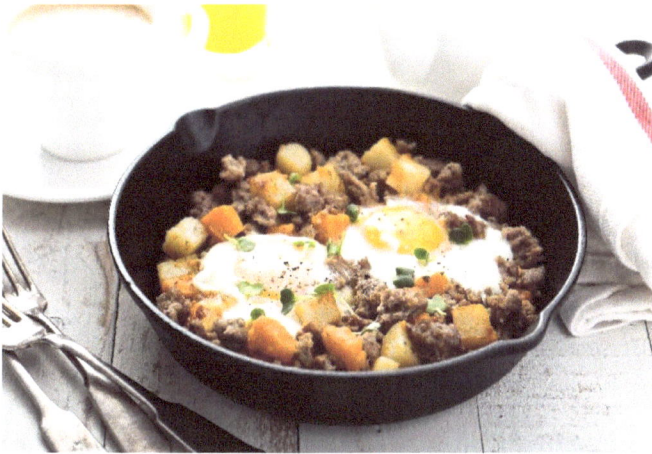

Servings: 4

Prep Time: 20 minutes

Cook Time: 15 minutes

Ingredients:

12 ounces grass-fed ground beef

1 teaspoon olive oil

4 cups chopped sweet potatoes

1 medium yellow onion, chopped

1 medium red pepper, chopped

4 large eggs

Salt and pepper

Instructions:

1. Heat an ovenproof skillet over medium-high heat.

2. Cook the ground beef until browned then spoon it into a bowl and drain the fat from the skillet.

3. Reheat the skillet over medium-high heat with the oil.

4. Add the sweet potatoes and cook without stirring for 3 to 4 minutes until the bottom starts to brown.

5. Stir the sweet potatoes and cook until they start to soften.

6. Preheat the oven to 400°F and increase the heat to high.

7. Add the onion and red pepper and cook for 4 to 5 minutes until the vegetables are softened.

8. Remove from heat then make four wells in the mixture.

9. Crack an egg into each well and season with salt and pepper.

10. Transfer to the oven and bake for 10 to 14 minutes until the eggs are set.

Turmeric Ginger Beet Juice

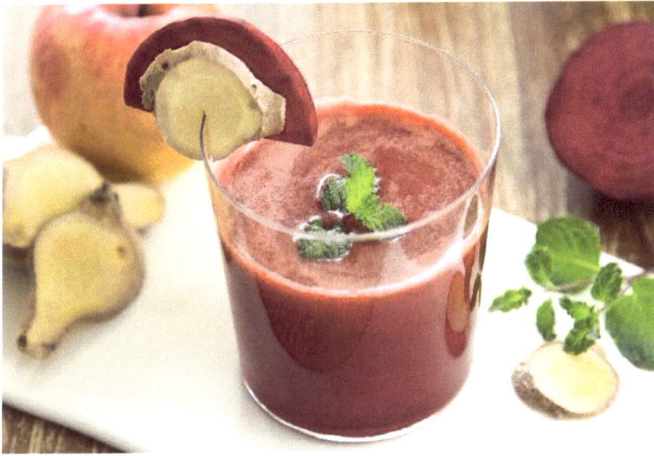

Servings: 1 to 2

Prep Time: 10 minutes

Cook Time: None

Ingredients:

- 2 medium red apples, cored
- 1 medium beet
- 3 leaves collard greens
- 2 leaves kale
- 1 small lemon
- 1 lime
- 1-inch piece of ginger root
- 1-inch piece of turmeric root

Instructions:

1. Clean the ingredients well and chop them to fit in a juicer.
2. Place a large glass or a container under the mouth of the juicer.
3. Feed the ingredients (except the flaxseed) through the juicer in the order listed.
4. Stir the flaxseed into the juice then enjoy immediately.

Cinnamon Banana Pancakes

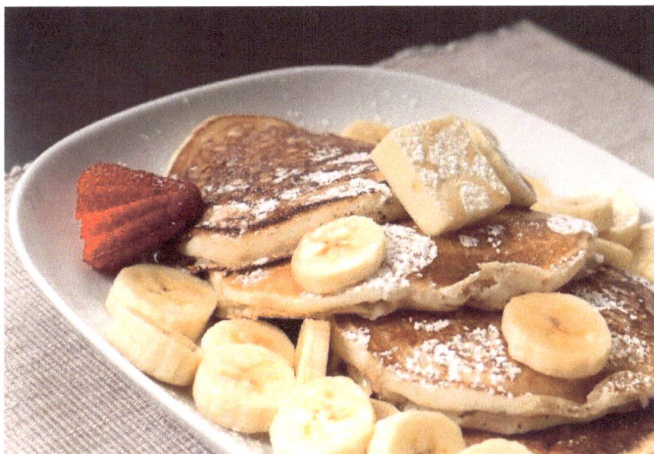

Servings: 1

Prep Time: 5 minutes

Cook Time: 10 minutes

Ingredients:

1 medium banana, very ripe, mashed

1 tablespoon coconut flour

1 tablespoon unsweetened almond milk

1 large egg

1/8 teaspoon baking powder

Pinch ground cinnamon

Instructions:

1. Combine the banana, coconut flour, almond milk, egg, baking powder and cinnamon in a mixing bowl.

2. Stir until well combined and preheat a skillet over medium heat.

3. Add the coconut oil and let it melt then spoon the batter into the skillet using about 2 tablespoons per pancake.

4. Cook until bubbles form in the surface of the batter then flip the pancakes.

5. Let them cook until the undersides are browned then remove to a plate.

6. Serve with sliced bananas and fresh strawberries.

Cranberry Flaxseed Protein Smoothie

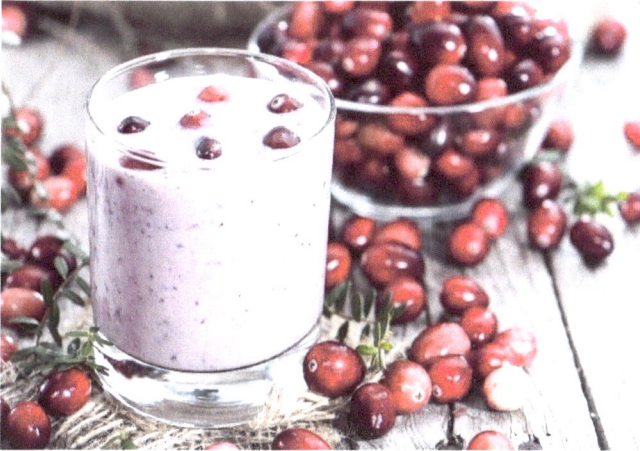

Servings: 1

Prep Time: 5 minutes

Cook Time: none

Ingredients:

1 cup frozen cranberries

1 cup unsweetened almond milk

1 small frozen banana

1 scoop egg white protein powder

2 tablespoons ground flaxseed

½ teaspoon vanilla extract

Liquid stevia, to taste

Instructions:

1. Combine the ingredients in a blender and pulse to chop.

2. Blend for 30 to 60 seconds on high speed until smooth.

3. Pour into a large glass and enjoy immediately.

Broccoli Kale Omelet

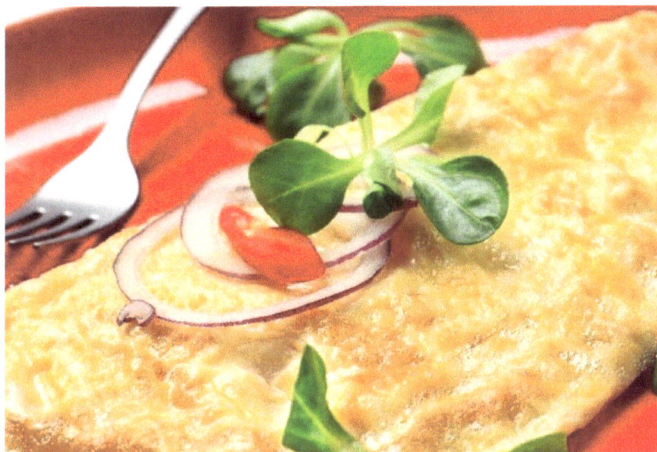

Servings: 1

Prep Time: 5 minutes

Cook Time: 10 minutes

Ingredients:

2 teaspoons olive oil, divided

½ cup diced broccoli

¼ cup diced yellow onion

½ cup chopped kale

1 clove minced garlic

3 large eggs

1 teaspoon fresh chopped chives

Salt and pepper

Instructions:

1. Heat 1 teaspoon oil in a small skillet over medium-high heat.
2. Add the broccoli and onion and cook until browned, about 4 minutes.
3. Stir in the kale and garlic and cook for 1 minute more, stirring often.
4. Spoon the veggies into a bowl and reheat the skillet with the remaining oil.
5. Whisk together the eggs, chives, salt and pepper and pour into the skillet.
6. Cook for 1 to 2 minutes without disturbing until the bottom starts to set.
7. Tilt the pan to spread the uncooked egg and cook 1 minute more.
8. Spoon the veggies over half the omelet and fold it over.
9. Cook until the eggs are set then slide onto a plate to serve.

Almond Sweet Potato Waffles

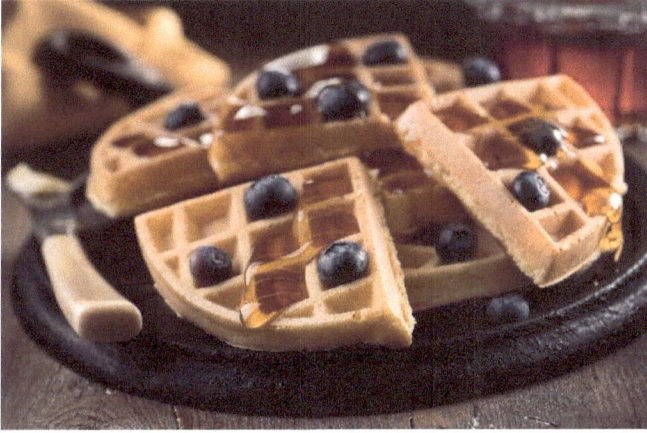

Servings: 4

Prep Time: 10 minutes

Cook Time: 15 minutes

Ingredients:

1 cup almond flour

2 ½ tablespoons coconut flour

1 teaspoon ground cinnamon

½ teaspoon baking soda

¼ teaspoon salt

½ cup cooked sweet potato, mashed

6 tablespoons unsweetened almond milk

2 large eggs, whisked

2 tablespoons honey

2 teaspoons vanilla extract

Instructions:

1. Whisk together the almond flour, coconut flour, cinnamon, baking soda, and salt in a mixing bowl.

2. In a separate bowl, whisk together the sweet potato, almond milk, eggs, honey, and vanilla.

3. Stir the wet ingredients into the dry until smooth and well combined.

4. Let the batter rest while you preheat the waffle iron.

5. Spoon the batter into the waffle iron and cook according to the directions.

Broccoli Apple Juice

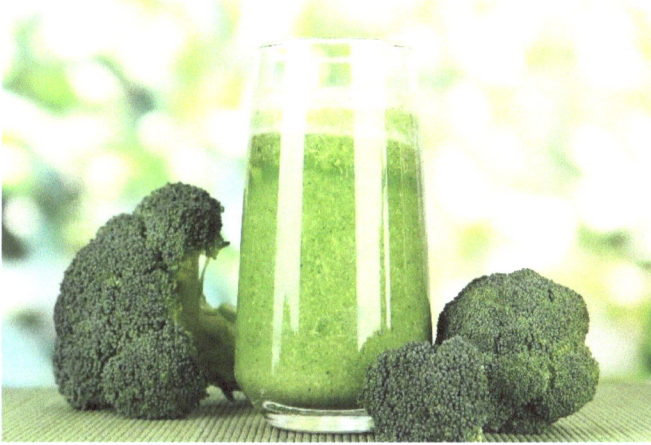

Servings: 1 to 2

Prep Time: 10 minutes

Cook Time: None

Ingredients:

2 medium green apples, cored

1 medium red apple, cored

1 small head broccoli

2 small tomatoes

1 small handful baby spinach

1 small lemon

1 lime

Instructions:

1. Clean the ingredients well and chop them to fit in a juicer.

2. Place a large glass or a container under the mouth of the juicer.

3. Feed the ingredients through the juicer in the order listed.

4. Stir the juice well then enjoy immediately.

Blueberry Pumpkin Seed Porridge

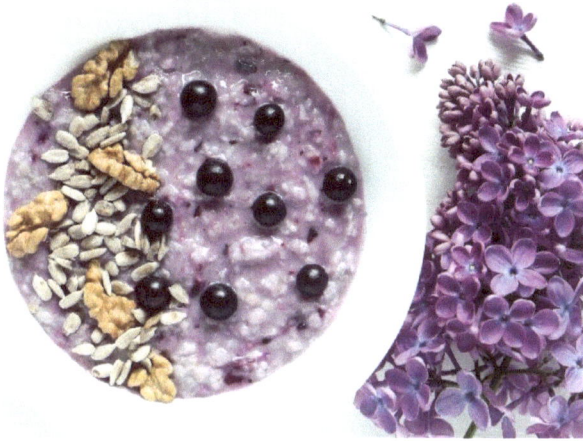

Servings: 2

Prep Time: 5 minutes

Cook Time: none

Ingredients:

¼ cup chopped pecans

2 tablespoons shredded unsweetened coconut

2 tablespoons flaxseed

1 tablespoon chia seeds

¼ teaspoon salt

1 cup boiling water

Instructions:

1. Combine the pecans, coconut, flaxseed, chia seeds, and salt in a food processor.

2. Pulse until finely ground then pour in the boiling water with the processor running on low speed.

3. Slowly increase the speed until the mixture is smooth then spoon into two bowls.

4. Serve with toasted walnuts, pumpkin seeds, and blueberries.

Spinach Green Apple Smoothie

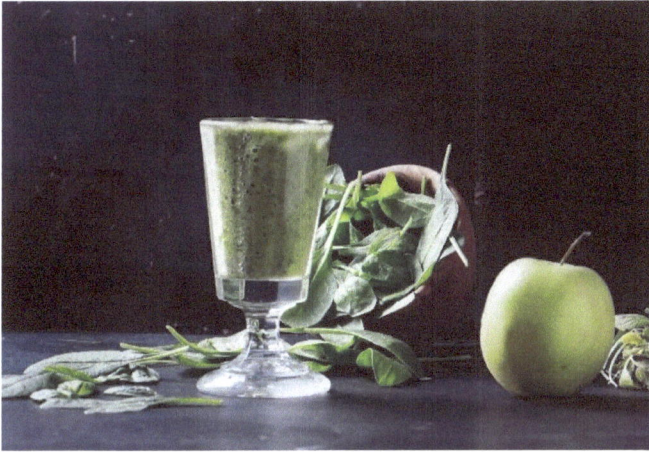

Servings: 1

Prep Time: 5 minutes

Cook Time: none

Ingredients:

1 cup fresh baby spinach

1 small green apple, cored and diced

¼ cup diced cucumber

1 cup unsweetened almond milk

½ cup ice cubes

2 tablespoons chia seeds

1 tablespoon fresh lemon juice

Liquid stevia, to taste

Instructions:

1. Combine the ingredients in a blender and pulse to chop.

2. Blend for 30 to 60 seconds on high speed until smooth.

3. Pour into a large glass and enjoy immediately.

Blueberry Flaxseed Muffins

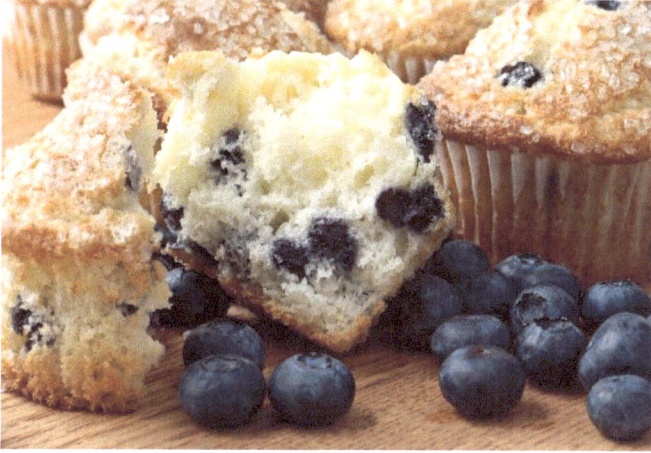

Servings: 10 to 12

Prep Time: 5 minutes

Cook Time: 25 minutes

Ingredients:

2 ¼ cups almond flour

¼ cup ground flaxseed

1 tablespoon coconut flour

½ teaspoon baking soda

¼ teaspoon salt

¼ cup unsweetened almond milk

¼ cup maple syrup

¼ cup melted coconut oil

2 teaspoons vanilla extract

2 large eggs

1 cup fresh blueberries

Instructions:

1. Preheat the oven to 350°F and line a muffin pan with paper liners.
2. Combine the almond flour, coconut flour, flaxseed, baking soda, and salt in a mixing bowl.
3. In a separate bowl, whisk together the almond milk, maple syrup, coconut oil, and vanilla.
4. Whisk in the eggs one at a time then stir the wet ingredients into the dry until smooth.
5. Fold in the blueberries then spoon the batter into the pan.
6. Bake for 22 to 25 minutes until a knife inserted in the center comes out clean.
7. Cool the muffins in the pan for 5 minutes then turn out.

Spinach and Herb Omelet

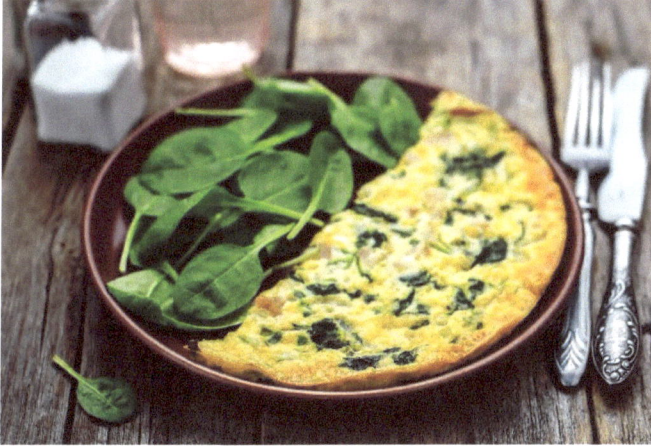

Servings: 1

Prep Time: 5 minutes

Cook Time: 10 minutes

Ingredients:

2 teaspoons olive oil, divided

1 cup fresh baby spinach

¼ cup diced yellow onion

1 clove minced garlic

3 large eggs

1 teaspoon fresh chopped chives

Salt and pepper

Instructions:

1. Heat 1 teaspoon oil in a small skillet over medium-high heat.

2. Add the spinach, onion, and garlic then cook until browned, about 4 minutes.

3. Spoon the veggies into a bowl and reheat the skillet with the remaining oil.

4. Whisk together the eggs, chives, salt and pepper and pour into the skillet.

5. Cook for 1 to 2 minutes without disturbing until the bottom starts to set.

6. Tilt the pan to spread the uncooked egg and cook 1 minute more.

7. Spoon the veggies over half the omelet and fold it over.

8. Cook until the eggs are set then slide onto a plate to serve.

Strawberry Coconut Smoothie

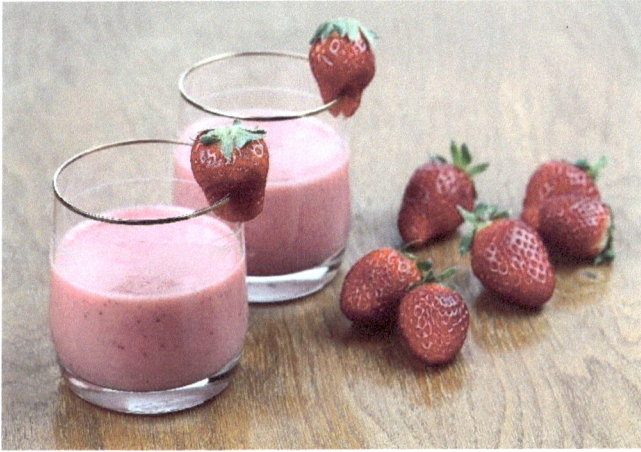

Servings: 1

Prep Time: 5 minutes

Cook Time: none

Ingredients:

1 cup frozen sliced strawberries

1 small frozen banana

1 cup unsweetened almond milk

¼ cup canned coconut milk

1 tablespoon chia seeds

¼ teaspoon vanilla extract

Liquid stevia, to taste

Instructions:

1. Combine the ingredients in a blender and pulse to chop.

2. Blend for 30 to 60 seconds on high speed until smooth.

3. Pour into a large glass and enjoy immediately.

Wild Mushroom Soup

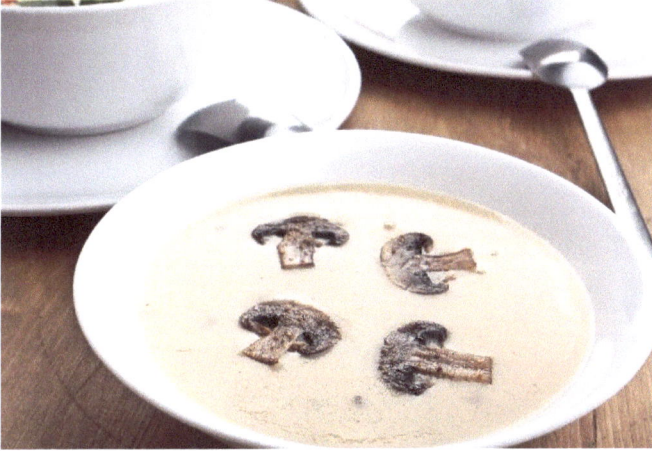

Servings: 4

Prep Time: 15 minutes

Cook Time: 15 minutes

Ingredients:

1 tablespoon olive oil

1 small yellow onion, chopped

1 ½ pounds sliced wild mushrooms

2 cloves minced garlic

1 tablespoon fresh chopped thyme

6 cups chicken broth

1 cup coconut milk

Salt and pepper

Instructions:

1. Heat the oil in a saucepan over medium-high heat.
2. Add the onions and sauté for 3 to 4 minutes until browned.
3. Stir in the mushrooms, garlic, and thyme and cook for 7 to 8 minutes until they release most of their liquid.
4. Add the chicken broth and bring to a boil.
5. Reduce heat and simmer for 15 minutes on medium-low.
6. Whisk in the coconut milk then season with salt and pepper to taste.
7. Simmer until thickened then serve hot.

Roasted Vegetable Quinoa Salad

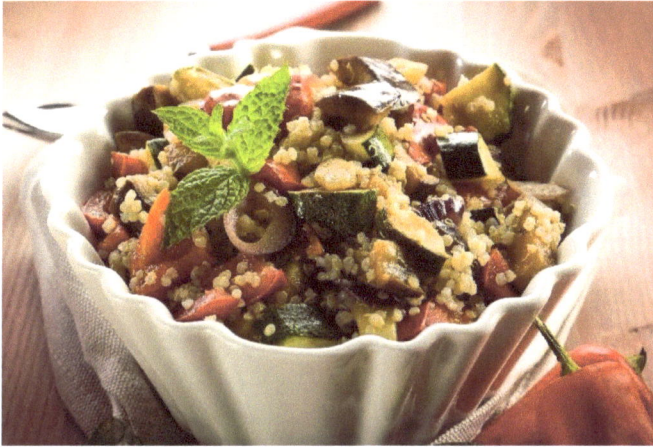

Servings: 4

Prep Time: 10 minutes

Cook Time: 15 minutes

Ingredients:

6 ounces diced mushrooms

1 medium yellow onion, chopped

1 small zucchini, diced

1 small red pepper, diced

1 small green pepper, diced

2 teaspoons fresh chopped rosemary

1 teaspoon minced garlic

Salt and pepper

3 tablespoons olive oil

½ cup quinoa, uncooked

¾ cup water

Instructions:

1. Preheat the oven to 400°F and line a baking sheet with foil.
2. Toss the veggies with olive oil, rosemary, garlic, salt and pepper then spread them evenly on the baking sheet.
3. Roast for 15 minutes, stirring halfway through.
4. Combine the quinoa and water in a saucepan and bring to boil.
5. Reduce heat and simmer for 15 minutes, covered.
6. Remove from heat and fluff with a fork then spoon into a large salad bowl to cool for a few minutes.
7. Toss in the roasted vegetables then serve warm.

Creamy Broccoli Spinach Soup

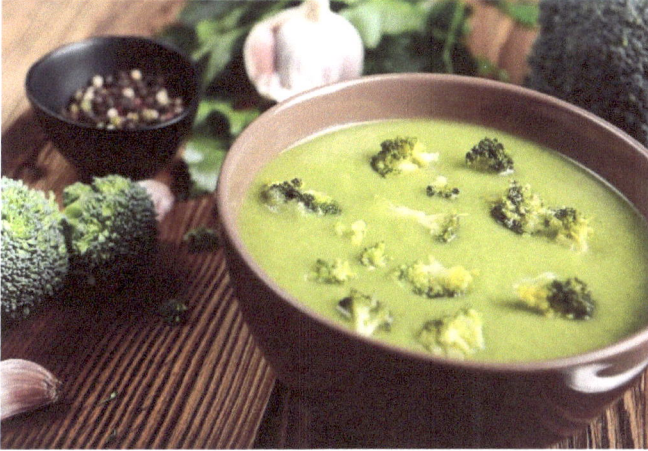

Servings: 4

Prep Time: 15 minutes

Cook Time: 10 minutes

Ingredients:

1 tablespoon olive oil

1 small yellow onion, chopped

2 cloves minced garlic

4 cups chopped broccoli

3 cups chicken broth

4 cups fresh baby spinach

2 tablespoons grated parmesan

Salt and pepper

¼ cup nonfat Greek yogurt, plain

Instructions:

1. Heat the oil in a saucepan over medium heat.
2. Add the onion and sauté for 3 minutes then stir in the garlic.
3. Cook for another 2 minutes until fragrant then add the broccoli.
4. Sauté for 10 minutes over medium heat until tender then stir in the chicken broth and bring to a boil.
5. Reduce heat and simmer for 10 minutes then remove from heat.
6. Stir in the spinach, parmesan cheese, salt, and pepper.
7. Puree the soup using an immersion blender then whisk in the yogurt.

Quinoa Tabbouleh Salad with Salmon

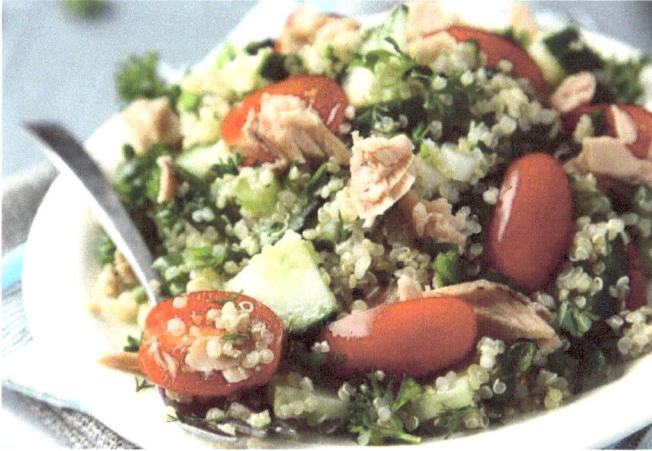

Servings: 6

Prep Time: 15 minutes

Cook Time: none

Ingredients:

1 ¼ cup water

1 cup uncooked quinoa

½ teaspoon salt

½ cup olive oil

3 tablespoons fresh lemon juice

1 clove minced garlic

Salt and pepper

1 English cucumber, quartered and sliced

2 cups cherry tomatoes, halved

¾ cup fresh chopped parsley

½ cup fresh chopped mint

¼ cup sliced scallions

Instructions:

1. Combine the water, quinoa, and salt in a saucepan and bring to a boil.
2. Reduce heat to medium-low and simmer, covered, for 10 minutes until the quinoa is tender then remove from heat and let stand.
3. Whisk together the olive oil, lemon juice, and garlic in a bowl and season with salt and pepper.
4. Spread the quinoa on a baking sheet to cool then spoon into a salad bowl.
5. Stir in about ¼ cup of the olive oil mixture then toss in the cucumber, tomatoes, parsley, scallions, and mint.
6. Drizzle with the remaining dressing to serve.

Mediterranean Couscous-Stuffed Peppers

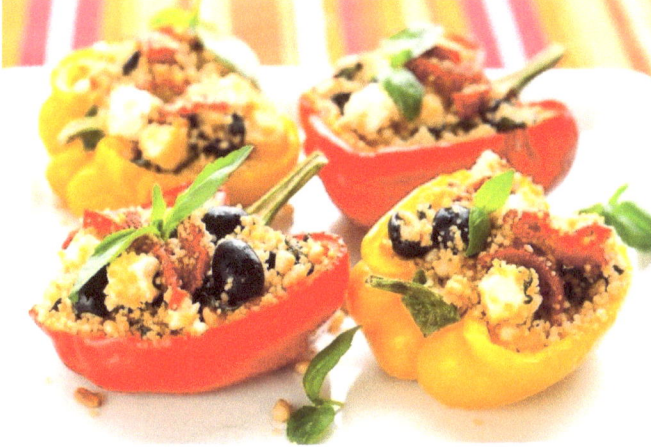

Servings: 6

Prep Time: 10 minutes

Cook Time: 25 minutes

Ingredients:

6 medium bell peppers

1 cup chicken broth

1 cup uncooked couscous

½ cup roasted red peppers, drained and chopped

½ cup diced yellow onion

3 cloves minced garlic

½ cup sliced black olives

Salt and pepper

1 cup crumbled feta cheese

½ cup water

Instructions:

1. Preheat the oven to 350°F.
2. Slice the tops off the peppers and remove the seeds and pith then place them in a casserole dish or glass baking dish.
3. Bring the chicken stock to boil in a small saucepan then stir in the couscous.
4. Remove from heat and cover for 5 minutes until the liquid is absorbed.
5. Spoon the couscous into a bowl and stir in the roasted red peppers, onion, garlic, and olives – season with salt and pepper to taste.
6. Spoon the mixture into the peppers and sprinkle with feta cheese.
7. Pour the water into the casserole dish around the peppers and cover with foil.
8. Bake for 25 minutes until tender then serve hot.

Vegan Cauliflower Chickpea Burgers

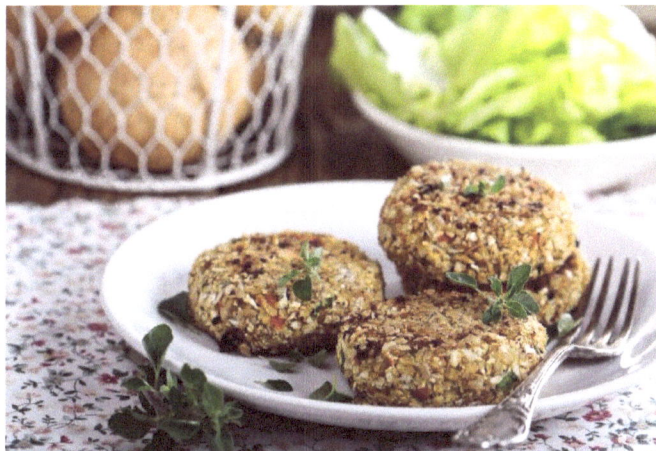

Servings: 4 to 6

Prep Time: 10 minutes

Cook Time: 45 minutes

Ingredients:

1 small head cauliflower, chopped

1 tablespoon olive oil

1 small yellow onion, chopped

½ small red pepper, diced

1 clove minced garlic

½ (15-ounce) can chickpeas, rinsed and drained

½ cup whole-wheat breadcrumbs

½ teaspoon ground cumin

¼ teaspoon turmeric

Salt and pepper

Instructions:

1. Preheat the oven to 375°F and line a baking sheet with foil.
2. Steam the cauliflower until very tender then drain and place in a bowl to cool.
3. Heat the oil in a skillet over medium-low heat then add the onion and pepper.
4. Sauté until tender, about 4 to 5 minutes, then stir in the garlic – cook 1 minute.
5. Place the chickpeas in a bowl and mash gently with a fork then add the cauliflower and mash it all together.
6. Stir in the onions, pepper, and garlic along with the remaining ingredients.
7. Shape the mixture into small patties then place them on the baking sheet.
8. Bake for 25 minutes then flip and bake another 20 minutes.

Vegetarian Lentil Tacos

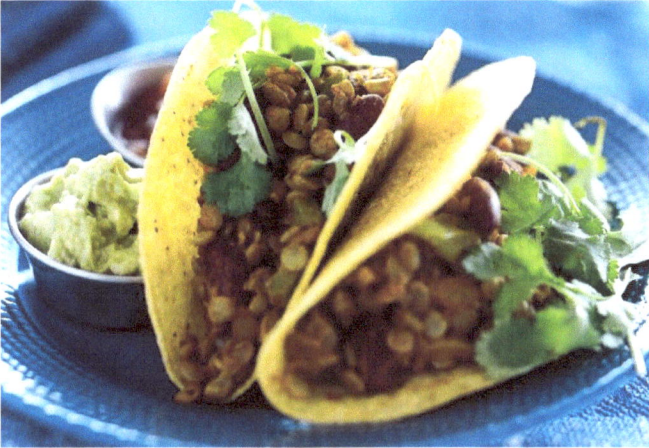

Servings: 4 to 5

Prep Time: 10 minutes

Cook Time: 20 minutes

Ingredients:

1 tablespoon olive oil

1 small yellow onion, chopped

1 cup dried brown lentils, picked over

2 tablespoons taco seasoning

1 tablespoon minced garlic

1 tablespoon tomato paste

2 cups vegetable broth

Instructions:

1. Heat the oil in a saucepan over medium heat then add the onion.
2. Sauté for 5 minutes until tender then stir in the lentils, taco seasoning, garlic, and tomato paste.
3. Cook for 1 minute, stirring often, then stir in the vegetable broth.
4. Bring to a boil then simmer, uncovered, for 10 minutes.
5. Reduce heat to low and simmer, covered, for 5 minutes until lentils are tender.
6. Spoon the lentil mixture into taco shells and serve with your favorite taco toppings.

Fried Vegetable Fritters

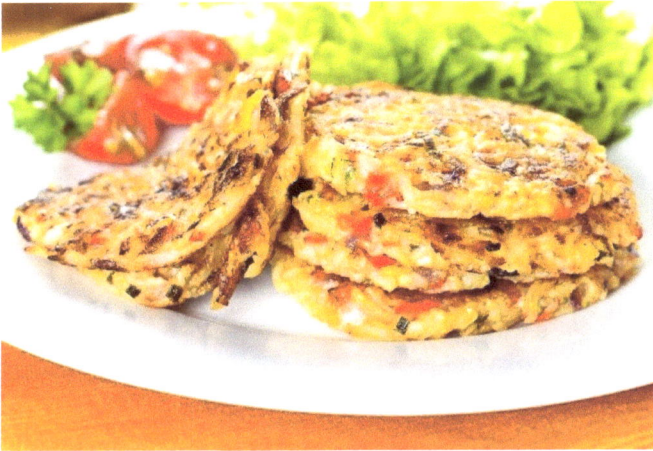

Servings: 4 to 6

Prep Time: 15 minutes

Cook Time: 15 minutes

Ingredients:

2 large carrots

2 medium sweet potatoes

2 small zucchinis

1 small yellow onion, minced

¼ cup fresh chopped parsley

½ cup almond flour

3 large eggs, separated

Salt and pepper

2 tablespoons olive oil

Instructions:

1. Grate the sweet potato, carrot, and zucchini into a bowl.
2. Stir in the onion, parsley, almond flour, egg yolks, salt and pepper.
3. Beat the egg whites to stiff peaks in a separate bowl then fold into the mixture.
4. Heat the oil in a large skillet over medium heat.
5. Scoop about 1/3 cup of the mixture into the skillet and cook for 5 minutes until the underside is lightly browned.
6. Flip the fritters and cook until browned on the other side.
7. Remove the fritters to paper towels to drain and repeat with remaining batter.

Sesame Shrimp and Veggie Stir-Fry

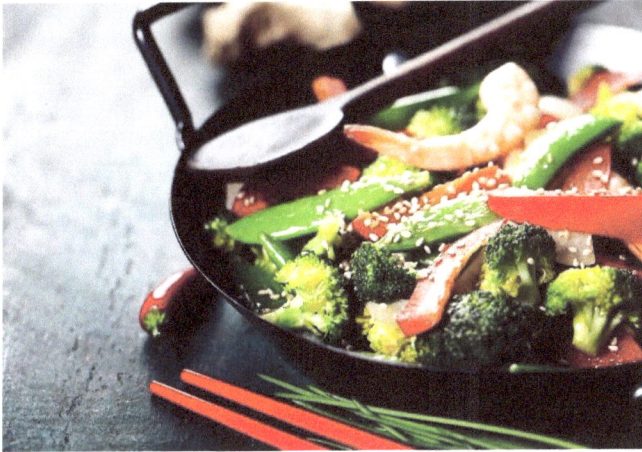

Servings: 4

Prep Time: 10 minutes

Cook Time: 20 minutes

Ingredients:

¼ cup soy sauce

3 tablespoons rice vinegar

1 tablespoon toasted sesame oil

½ teaspoon sriracha

1 tablespoon cornstarch

2 tablespoons olive oil

12 ounces chopped broccoli florets

2 medium carrots, sliced

1 large red pepper, sliced

1 cup snow peas

2 tablespoons grated ginger

1 tablespoon minced garlic

1 pound uncooked shrimp, peeled and deveined

Instructions:

1. Whisk together the soy sauce, rice vinegar, sesame oil, sriracha, and cornstarch in a small bowl then set aside.

2. Heat the oil in a large skillet over medium-high heat.

3. Add the broccoli and cook for 5 to 6 minutes until tender-crisp.

4. Stir in the carrots, peppers, and snow peas and cook for 2 minutes.

5. Stir in the garlic and ginger and sauté for 1 minute then push all of the vegetables to the sides of the skillet.

6. Add the shrimp and cook for 1 to 2 minutes until just opaque.

7. Spoon a few tablespoons of water into the skillet to loosen the browned bits then stir-fry everything together with the sauce.

8. Simmer until the sauce thickens then serve over steamed brown rice.

Pepper-Crusted Seared Ribeye

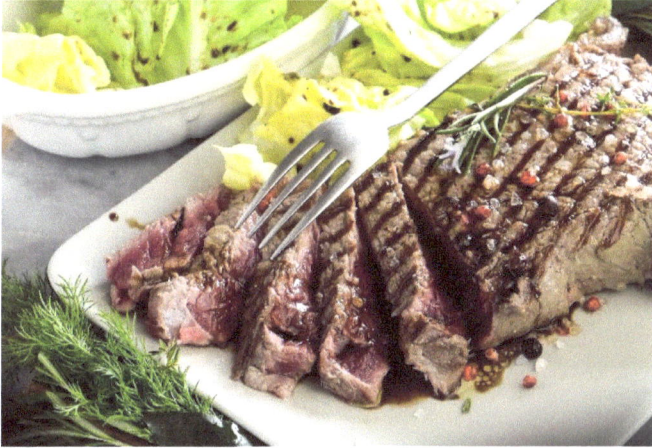

Servings: 4

Prep Time: 5 minutes

Cook Time: 10 minutes

Ingredients:

4 (6- to 8-ounce) ribeye steaks, 1 ½ inches thick

¼ cup brown mustard

¼ cup crushed black peppercorns

2 tablespoons fresh cracked pepper

Salt to taste

Instructions:

1. Brush the steak with mustard then sprinkle with crushed peppercorns and fresh-cracked pepper and salt.

2. Preheat the grill and grease the grates with olive oil cooking spray.

3. Place the steaks on the grill and cook for 3 to 4 minutes on each side for rare.

4. Transfer to a cutting board and let rest 5 minutes before slicing to serve.

Herb-Grilled Turkey Burgers

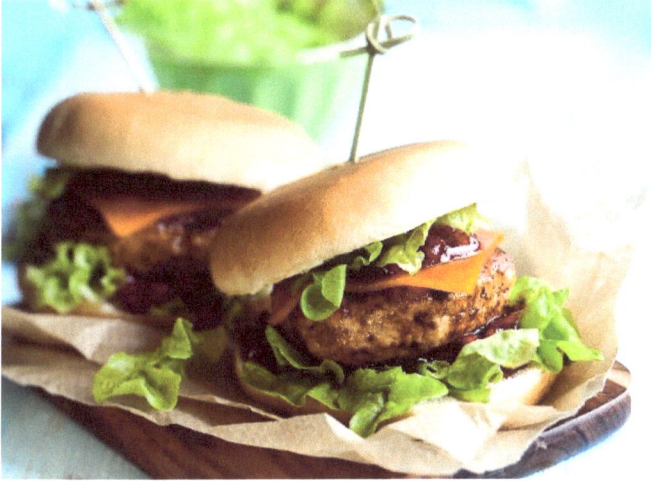

Servings: 4

Prep Time: 10 minutes

Cook Time: 12 minutes

Ingredients:

1 tablespoon olive oil

1 small yellow onion, chopped

2 cloves minced garlic

1-pound lean ground turkey

¼ cup fresh chopped parsley

2 teaspoons fresh chopped rosemary

1 ½ teaspoons fresh chopped sage

Salt and pepper

Instructions:

1. Heat the oil in a skillet over medium heat.
2. Add the onion and cook for 3 minutes then stir in the garlic and cook for another 2 minutes until fragrant.
3. Remove from heat and spoon into a large mixing bowl.
4. Stir in the ground turkey, herbs, salt and pepper until well combined.
5. Shape into four even-sized patties then preheat the grill.
6. Grease the grates with cooking spray then add the burger patties.
7. Cook for 5 to 6 minutes on each side until the internal temperature is 165°F.
8. Serve the burgers hot on toasted sandwich buns with your favorite toppings.

Grilled Salmon with Mango Sauce

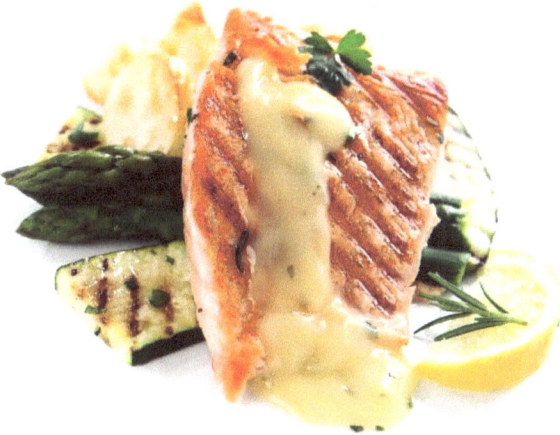

Servings: 4

Prep Time: 5 minutes

Cook Time: 15 minutes

Ingredients:

1 teaspoon garlic powder

1 teaspoon chili powder

Salt and pepper

1 large ripe mango, pitted and chopped

¼ cup canned coconut milk

2 tablespoons fresh cilantro

1 tablespoon fresh lemon juice

Instructions:

1. Combine the garlic powder, chili powder, salt and pepper in a small bowl.
2. Rub the spice mixture into the salmon.
3. Preheat a grill and grease the grates with olive oil cooking spray.
4. Add the salmon fillets and grill for 6 to 8 minutes on each side.
5. Combine the remaining ingredients in a food processor and blend smooth.
6. Serve the salmon hot drizzled with mango sauce.

Roasted Rosemary Chicken with Veggies

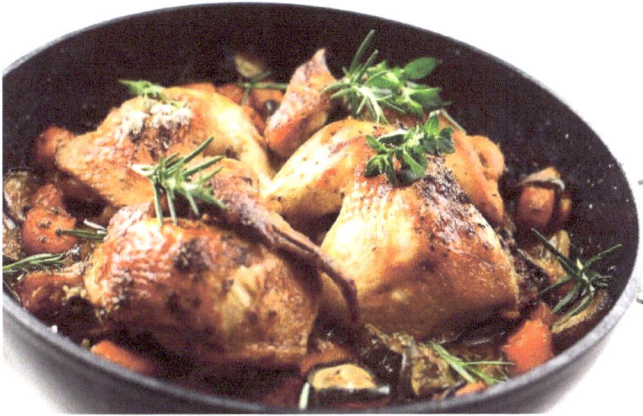

Servings: 4 to 6

Prep Time: 10 minutes

Cook Time: 1 hour

Ingredients:

2 tablespoons olive oil

2 pounds bone-in chicken legs

Salt and pepper

2 medium sweet potatoes, cut into chunks

1 large zucchini, sliced thick

1 large yellow onion, chopped

1 large carrot, peeled and sliced

1 cup chopped tomatoes

1 tablespoon fresh chopped rosemary

1 teaspoon fresh chopped thyme

Instructions:

1. Preheat the oven to 400°F.
2. Heat the oil in a large skillet over medium-high heat.
3. Season the chicken with salt and pepper then add to the skillet – cook until browned on all sides.
4. Toss the vegetables with another tablespoon or two of oil along with the rosemary, thyme, salt and pepper.
5. Spread the vegetables in a large glass baking dish and place the chicken skin-side down on top.
6. Roast for 30 minutes then turn the chicken and roast until cooked through, about another 25 to 30 minutes.

Garlic Herb Pork Tenderloin

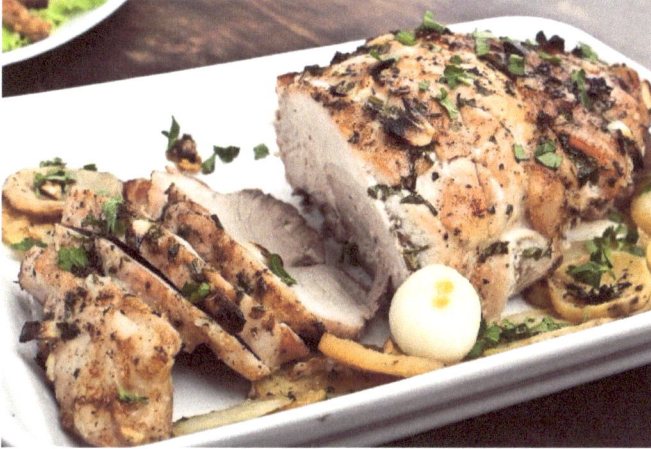

Servings: 4

Prep Time: 10 minutes

Cook Time: 45 minutes

Ingredients:

1 tablespoon minced garlic

1 teaspoon dried rosemary

1 teaspoon dried thyme

1 teaspoon dried basil

1 to 2 tablespoons olive oil

Salt and pepper

1 ¼ pounds boneless pork tenderloin

Instructions:

1. Preheat the oven to 425°F and line a baking sheet with foil.

2. Combine the garlic and herbs in a food processor and pulse in the oil to form a thick paste.

3. Season with salt and pepper then rub the mixture into the pork.

4. Place the pork on the baking sheet and roast for 35 to 45 minutes until the internal temperature reaches 145°F.

5. Remove the pork to a cutting board and let rest 5 to 10 minutes before slicing.

Halibut with Mango Salsa

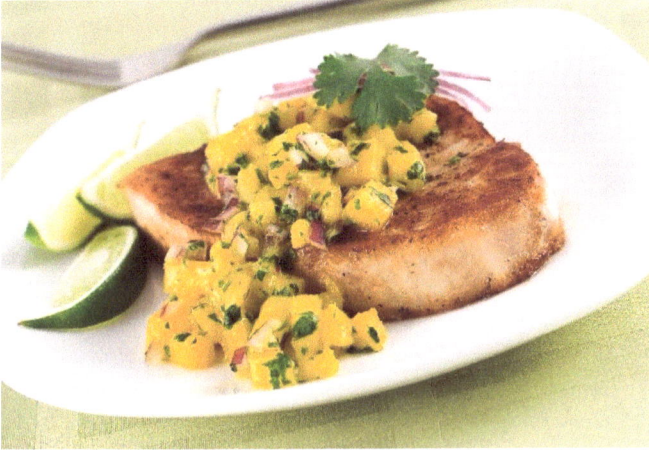

Servings: 4

Prep Time: 5 minutes

Cook Time: 15 minutes

Ingredients:

4 (6-ounce) boneless halibut fillets

1 tablespoon olive oil

Salt and pepper

2 tablespoons fresh chopped parsley

1 medium mango, pitted and diced

¼ cup diced red onion

2 tablespoons fresh chopped cilantro

1 tablespoon fresh lemon juice

Instructions:

1. Preheat the oven to 400°F and line a baking sheet with foil.
2. Brush the halibut with oil and season with salt and pepper.
3. Sprinkle with parsley then bake for 12 to 15 minutes until just cooked through.
4. Combine the remaining ingredients in a food processor and pulse until finely chopped.
5. Serve the halibut topped with the mango salsa with lime wedges on the side.

Herb Roasted Lamb Chops

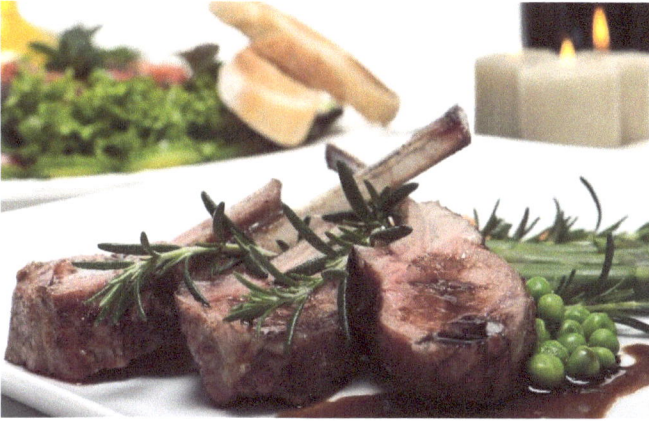

Servings: 4

Prep Time: 35 minutes

Cook Time: 15 minutes

Ingredients:

1 tablespoon olive oil

1 tablespoon minced garlic

1 tablespoon fresh chopped rosemary

1 tablespoon fresh chopped thyme

Salt and pepper

8 bone-in lamb chops

Instructions:

1. Combine the olive oil, garlic, rosemary, and thyme in a small bowl.

2. Season the lamb with salt and pepper then add it to a shallow dish.

3. Pour the herb mixture over it and turn to coat – let rest 30 minutes.

4. Preheat the oven to 400°F.

5. Grease a skillet with cooking spray and heat over high heat.

6. Add the lamb and cook for 2 to 3 minutes until browned on both sides.

7. Transfer the skillet to the oven and bake for 10 minutes.

8. Remove to a platter and let the lamb rest 5 minutes before serving.

Maple Roasted Brussels Sprouts

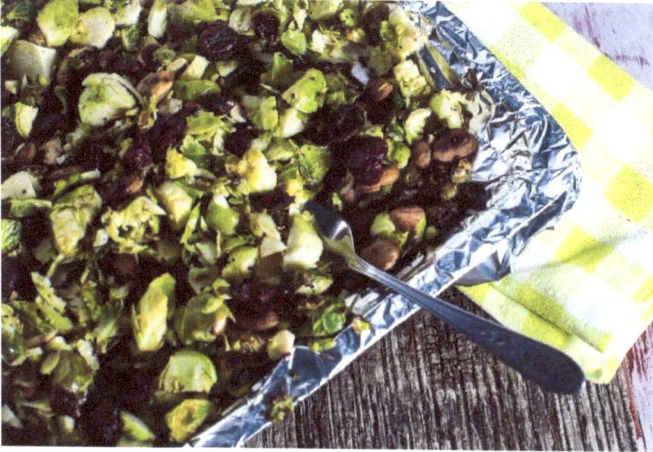

Servings: 4 to 6

Prep Time: 15 minutes

Cook Time: 35 minutes

Ingredients:

1 ½ pounds brussels sprouts

2 to 3 tablespoons olive oil

Salt and pepper

2 to 3 tablespoons maple syrup

Instructions:

1. Preheat the oven to 400°F and line a baking sheet with foil.

2. Trim the brussels sprouts and cut them in half.

3. Toss the brussels sprouts with oil, salt and pepper then spread on the baking sheet in a single layer.

4. Roast for 15 minutes then stir and roast another 10 minutes.

5. Drizzle with maple syrup then stir to coat and roast and other 10 minutes.

6. Transfer to a serving bowl and stir in the cranberries to serve.

Herb Roasted Root Veggies

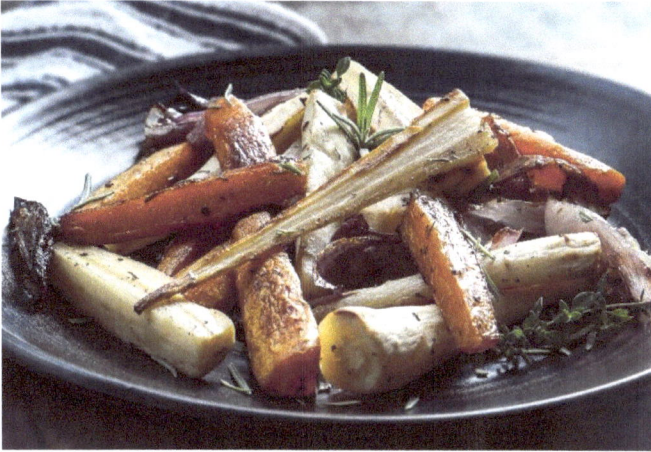

Servings: 4 to 6

Prep Time: 10 minutes

Cook Time: 20 minutes

Ingredients:

¾ pound carrots, sliced into sticks

½ pound parsnips, sliced into sticks

1 ½ pounds sweet potatoes, cut into wedges

Salt and pepper

3 tablespoons olive oil

2 teaspoons fresh chopped rosemary

1 teaspoon fresh chopped thyme

Instructions:

1. Preheat the oven to 450°F and line a baking sheet with foil.

2. Place the carrots and parsnips in a large saucepan and cover with cold water.

3. Add salt then cover and bring to a boil over high heat.

4. Reduce heat and simmer for 7 minutes then drain well then toss with oil, salt and pepper.

5. Spread on the baking dish and sprinkle with rosemary and thyme.

6. Roast for 20 minutes until tender then serve hot.

Garlic White Bean Hummus

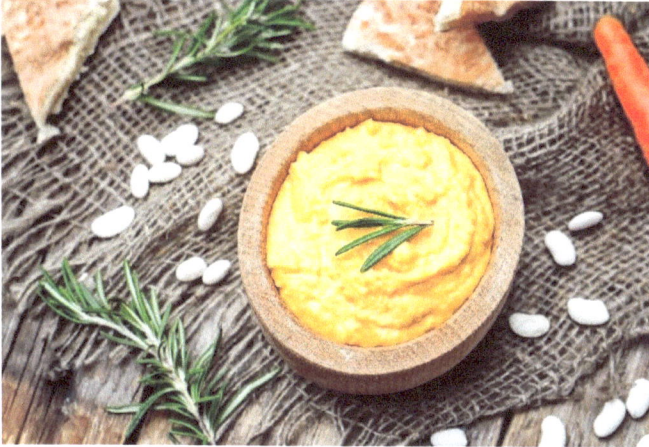

Servings: 4

Prep Time: 10 minutes

Cook Time: none

Ingredients:

1 (15-ounce) can white cannellini beans, rinsed and drained

2 tablespoons tahini

2 tablespoons olive oil

Juice from 1 lemon

½ teaspoon garlic powder

½ teaspoon onion powder

Salt and pepper

Instructions:

1. Combine the ingredients in a food processor and blend until smooth.
2. Check the consistency then blend in some water a tablespoon at a time to thin it, if needed.
3. Adjust seasoning to taste and serve with sliced veggies for dipping.

Baked Kale Chips

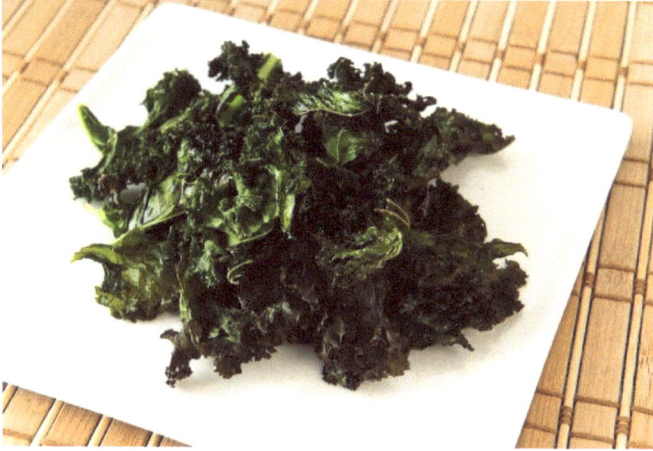

Servings: 4

Prep Time: 10 minutes

Cook Time: 25 minutes

Ingredients:

1 large bunch fresh kale

2 tablespoons olive oil

Salt and pepper

Instructions:

1. Preheat the oven to 400°F and line a baking sheet with parchment.

2. Rinse the kale well and shake dry then pat with paper towels to remove water.

3. Cut away the thick stems and tear the kale into 2-inch chunks.

4. Toss the kale with olive oil, salt, and pepper then spread on the baking sheet.

5. Bake for 15 minutes then turn the pan and bake another 5 to 10 minutes.

6. Remove from the oven and let cool until crisp then enjoy.

Cucumber Spinach Dip

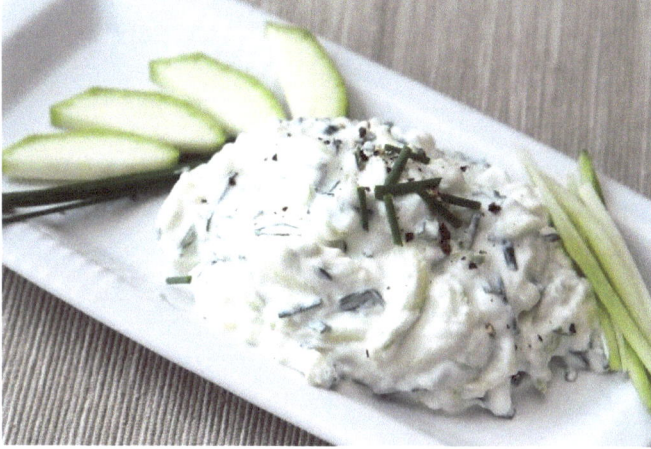

Servings: 6 to 8

Prep Time: 15 minutes

Cook Time: None

Ingredients:

½ cup canned coconut milk

3 tablespoons fresh lemon juice

2 tablespoons ground flaxseed

1 tablespoon coconut oil

Salt and pepper

1 teaspoon apple cider vinegar

1 small seedless cucumber, diced

1 handful fresh spinach, chopped

Instructions:

1. Combine the coconut milk, lemon juice, flaxseed, and coconut oil in a food processor.
2. Blend until smooth and well combined.
3. Season with salt and pepper to taste then blend in the apple cider vinegar.
4. Add the cucumber, spinach, cilantro, and dill.
5. Pulse several times to chop the cucumber and spinach.
6. Adjust seasoning to taste and serve with veggie slices for dipping.

Black Bean Brownies

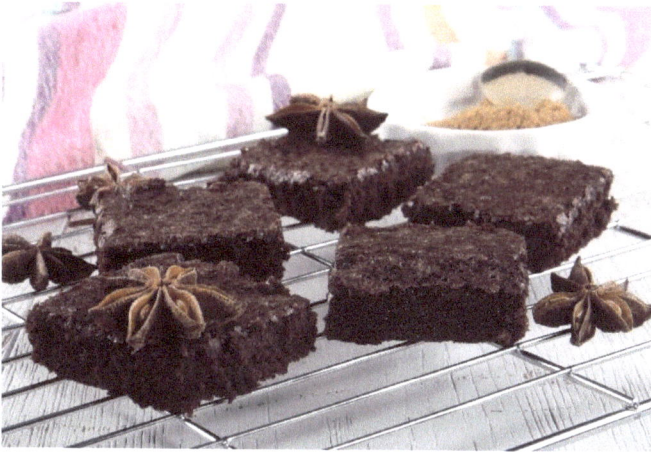

Servings: 9 to 12

Prep Time: 10 minutes

Cook Time: 20 minutes

Ingredients:

1 (15-ounce) can black beans, rinsed and drained

½ cup old-fashioned oats

4 to 6 tablespoons pure maple syrup

¼ cup coconut oil

1 tablespoon vanilla extract

½ teaspoon baking powder

¼ teaspoon salt

½ cup dark chocolate chips

Instructions:

1. Preheat the oven to 350°F and line a square baking pan with parchment.

2. Combine the black beans, oats, maple syrup, and coconut oil in a food processor and pulse several times.

3. Add the vanilla, baking powder and salt then blend until smooth and adjust sweetness to taste.

4. Spread the batter in the prepared pan and sprinkle with dark chocolate chips.

5. Bake for 16 to 20 minutes until the center is set.

6. Let the brownies cool completely before cutting into squares to serve.

Cherry Chia Pudding

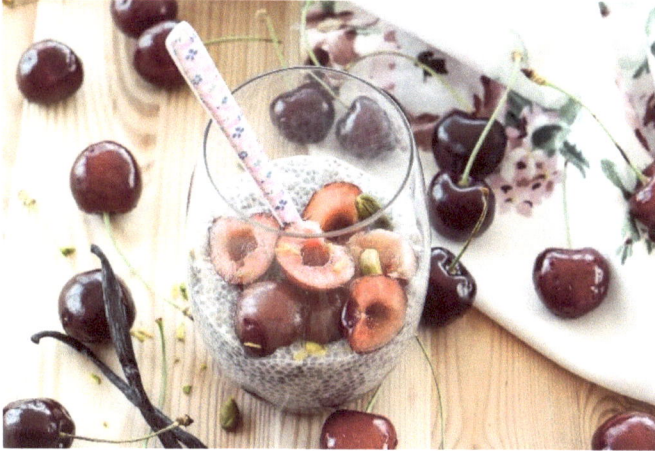

Servings: 4

Prep Time: 10 minutes

Cook Time: None

Ingredients:

1 (14-ounce) can coconut milk

3 to 4 tablespoons pure maple syrup

1 teaspoon almond extract

½ teaspoon vanilla extract

Pinch salt

3 cups fresh cherries, pitted and sliced

¾ cup chia seeds

½ cup ground flaxseed

Instructions:

1. Combine the coconut milk, maple syrup, almond extract, and vanilla extract in a blender with a pinch of salt.

2. Blend until well combined then add 2 cups cherries and blend smooth.

3. Pulse in the chia seeds and flaxseed.

4. Spoon the pudding into cups and chill for 1 hour.

5. Serve the pudding cold topped with the remaining cherries.

Avocado Chocolate Mousse

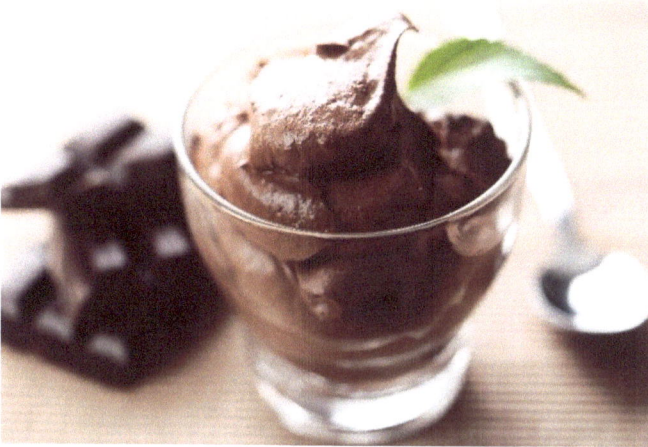

Servings: 4

Prep Time: 10 minutes

Cook Time: None

Ingredients:

4 ounces dark chocolate chips

2 large avocados, pitted and chopped

¼ cup unsweetened almond milk

3 tablespoons unsweetened cocoa powder

1 ½ teaspoons vanilla extract

Pinch salt

Instructions:

1. Melt the dark chocolate chips in the microwave and stir smooth.

2. Spoon the avocadoes into a food processor.

3. Add the almond milk, cocoa powder, vanilla, and salt and blend smooth.

4. Pour in the melted chocolate and blend until smooth and creamy, scraping down the bowl as needed.

5. Sweeten with liquid stevia to taste then spoon into cups.

6. Chill for 2 hours for a thicker mousse then serve cold.

Cocoa-Dusted Almonds

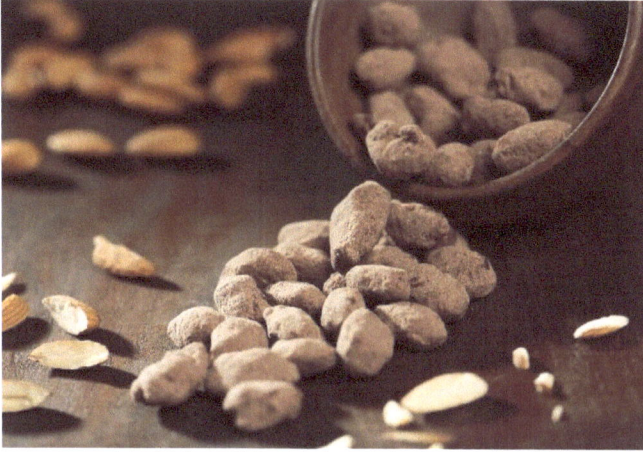

Servings: 6 to 8

Prep Time: 5 minutes

Cook Time: 10 minutes

Ingredients:

2 cups whole almonds, raw

2 tablespoons honey

1 ½ teaspoons salt

2 tablespoons unsweetened cocoa powder

Instructions:

1. Preheat the oven to 350°F and line a baking
   sheet with parchment.

2. Toss the almonds with the honey and salt, stirring to coat.

3. Spread in a single layer on the baking sheet.

4. Bake the almonds for 10 minutes, stirring once or twice to prevent burning.

5. Immediately return the almonds to the bowl and toss with the cocoa powder.

6. Let cool then store in an airtight container.

Flourless Almond Butter Cookies

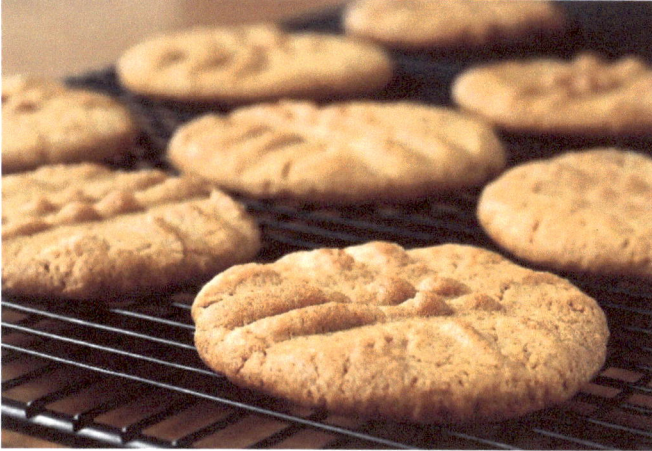

Servings: 16

Prep Time: 10 minutes

Cook Time: 10 minutes

Ingredients:

1 cup almond butter

¾ cup organic cane sugar, packed

1 large egg

1 teaspoon vanilla extract

1 teaspoon baking soda

Pinch salt

Instructions:

1. Preheat the oven to 350°F and line a baking sheet with parchment paper.

2. Combine the almond butter and sugar in a food processor.

3. Blend until smooth then add the egg and vanilla extract then pulse a few times.

4. Add the baking soda and sea salt then blend well.

5. Pinch off pieces of dough and roll them into balls then place them on the baking sheet about 2 inches apart.

6. Bake for 8 to 10 minutes until the cookies are just browned on the edges.

7. Let the cookies cool for 3 minutes then remove to a wire rack.

Gluten-Free Berry Crisp

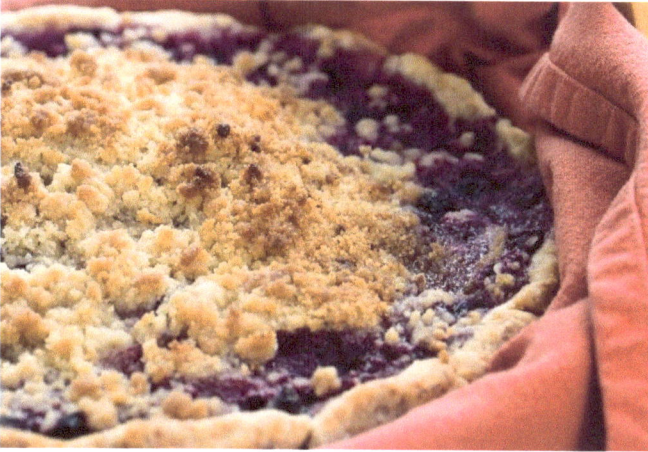

Servings: 6 to 8

Prep Time: 5 minutes

Cook Time: 45 minutes

Ingredients:

7 cups fresh mixed berries

2 to 3 tablespoons pure maple syrup

2 tablespoons arrowroot powder

1 tablespoon fresh lemon juice

1 cup almond flour

¾ cup shredded unsweetened coconut

1 cup chopped walnuts

½ cup coconut sugar

½ teaspoon salt

¼ cup coconut oil

Instructions:

1. Preheat the oven to 350°F and grease a glass pie plate.
2. Toss the berries with the maple syrup, arrowroot powder, and lemon juice then spread evenly in the pie plate.
3. Combine the almond flour, coconut, walnuts, coconut sugar, and salt in a mixing bowl and stir well.
4. Cut in the coconut oil until it forms a crumbled mixture then spread it over the berries in the pie plate.
5. Bake for 40 to 45 minutes until the top is browned and the fruit bubbling.
6. Cool for 10 minutes before serving.

Vegan Carrot Cake Cupcakes

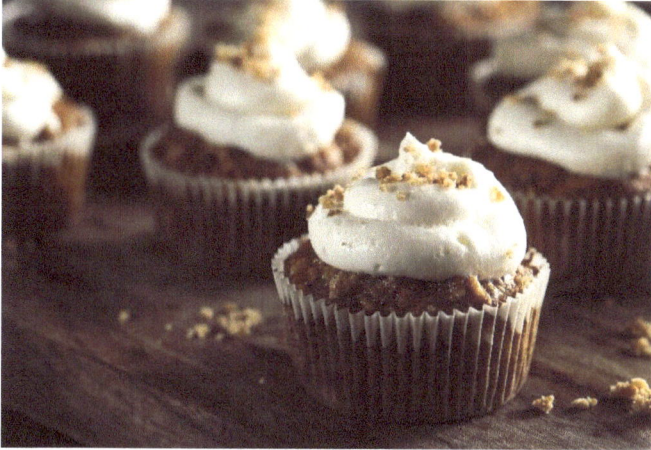

Servings: 9

Prep Time: 10 minutes

Cook Time: 25 minutes

Ingredients:

2 tablespoons ground flaxseed

6 tablespoons warm water

1 1/3 cup whole-wheat flour

1 teaspoon baking powder

¾ teaspoon baking soda

¾ teaspoon ground cinnamon

¼ teaspoon ground ginger

Pinch salt

¾ cup coconut sugar

½ cup olive oil

2 tablespoons unsweetened almond milk

2 teaspoons vanilla extract

2/3 cup grated carrot

Instructions:

1. Preheat the oven to 325°F and line 9 cups of a muffin pan with paper liners.
2. Combine the flaxseed and water in a blender – blend then set aside.
3. Whisk together the flour, baking powder, baking soda, cinnamon, ginger, and salt in a mixing bowl.
4. In a separate bowl, whisk together the coconut sugar, olive oil, almond milk, and vanilla extract with the flax mixture.
5. Stir the wet and dry ingredients together until well combined.
6. Fold in the carrots then spoon into the prepared pan, filling the cups 2/3 full.
7. Bake for 22 to 25 minutes until a knife inserted in the center comes out clean.

8 . Let the cupcakes cool completely then frost as desired.

Conclusion

The human body is a complex network of organs and systems that must remain in balance for good health. When something is thrown off, such as hormone levels, it can wreak all kinds of havoc on your health.

Estrogen is a hormone primarily responsible for female sex characteristics in women, but it can be found in men as well. In order for estrogen to do its job well without causing any problems, it needs to be balanced with another hormone – progesterone. When your estrogen-progesterone ratio becomes unbalanced, it leads to estrogen dominance and a variety of related symptoms.

Though hormone therapy is an option for low levels of estrogen, reducing estrogen levels can sometimes be tricky. Making healthy changes to your diet and lifestyle is the best way to reduce estrogen naturally without any negative consequences. In reading this book, you've received some valuable information about how to do that. All that is left now is for you to put that advice into action.

So, take to heart what you've learned here about estrogen dominance and its link to conditions like uterine fibroids and Hashimoto's. Use that knowledge to make improvements in your life, starting with some of the tasty recipes we've provided. Good luck!

References

"7 Foods for Lowering Estrogen Levels in Men." Healthline. <https://www.healthline.com/health/low-testosterone/anti-estrogen-diet-men>

"8 Surprising High-Estrogen Symptoms in Men." UHN Daily. <https://universityhealthnews.com/daily/nutrition/8-surprising-high-estrogen-symptoms-in-men/>

Aragon, Britta. "15 Ways to Protect Yourself from Excess Estrogen." Daily Dose Blog. <https://www.bewell.com/blog/15-ways-to-protect-yourself-from-excess-estrogen/>

Black, Brandi. "Signs of Estrogen Dominance & 5 Ways to Decrease Symptoms." Paleo Hacks. <https://blog.paleohacks.com/estrogen-dominance/#>

"Environmental Estrogens." Energetic Nutrition. <https://www.energeticnutrition.com/vitalzym/xeno_phyto_estrogens.html>

"Epidemic Disease Occurrence." CDC. <https://www.cdc.gov/ophss/csels/dsepd/ss1978/lesson1/section11.html>

"Estrogen Dominance in Men." World Health Net.
<https://www.worldhealth.net/news/estrogen-dominance-men-ruining-your-health-/>

"Estrogen and Progesterone: Two Important Hormones."
Taylor Medical.
<https://taylormedicalgroup.net/hormones/estrogen-and-progesterone>

"Estrogen and Your Thyroid." Healthful Elements.
<https://www.healthfulelements.com/blog/2013/01/estrogen-and-your-thyroid>

"Estrogen Levels in Men." BodyLogicMD.
<https://www.bodylogicmd.com/hormones-for-men/estrogen>

"Fibroids." UCLA Health. <http://obgyn.ucla.edu/fibroids>

"Hashimoto's Disease." Mayo Clinic.
<https://www.mayoclinic.org/diseases-conditions/hashimotos-disease/diagnosis-treatment/drc-20351860>

"High-Estrogen Foods to Avoid + Environmental Estrogens
Hiding in Your Home." Dr. Axe. <https://draxe.com/5-high-estrogen-foods-avoid/

"Hypothyroidism (Underactive Thyroid)." Mayo Clinic.
<https://www.mayoclinic.org/diseases-conditions/hypothyroidism/symptoms-causes/syc-

20350284>

Nothrup, Christiane. "What Are the Symptoms of Estrogen Dominance?" Christiane Nothrup, M.D. <https://www.drnorthrup.com/estrogen-dominance/>

Sargis, Robert. "An Overview of the Ovaries: Estrogen, Progesterone, and Reproduction." Endocrine Web. <https://www.endocrineweb.com/endocrinology/overview-ovaries>

"Thyroid Gland." You and Your Hormones. <http://www.yourhormones.info/glands/thyroid-gland/>

"Uterine Fibroids." Mayo Clinic. <https://www.mayoclinic.org/diseases-conditions/uterine-fibroids/symptoms-causes/syc-20354288>

Wentz, Izabella. "Estrogen Dominance as a Trigger for Hashimoto's." Thyroid Pharmacist. <https://thyroidpharmacist.com/articles/estrogen-dominance-as-a-hashimotos-trigger/>

"What is Progesterone?" Hormone Health Network. <https://www.hormone.org/hormones-and-health/hormones/progesterone>

www.ingramcontent.com/pod-product-compliance
Lightning Source LLC
Chambersburg PA
CBHW041712200326
41518CB00005B/192